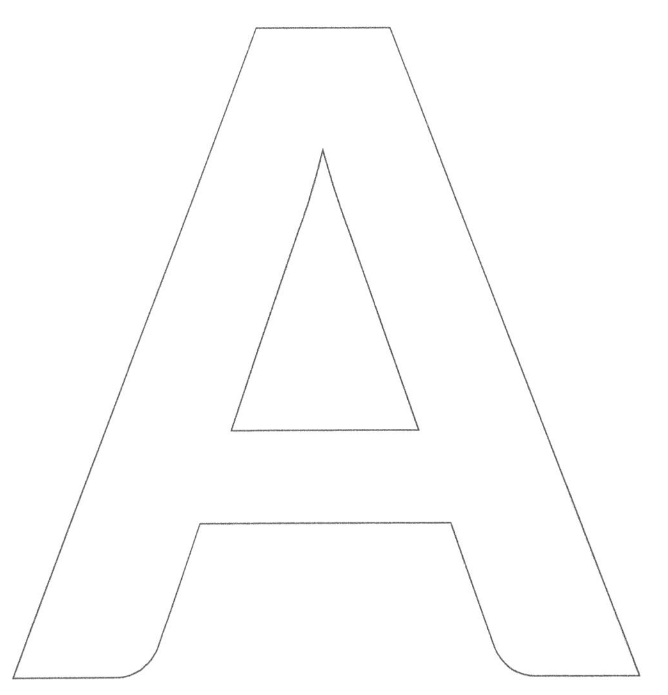

"You can do it. Get the ball rolling right now."

I will ACHIEVE

I will ACHIEVE

I will ACHIEVE

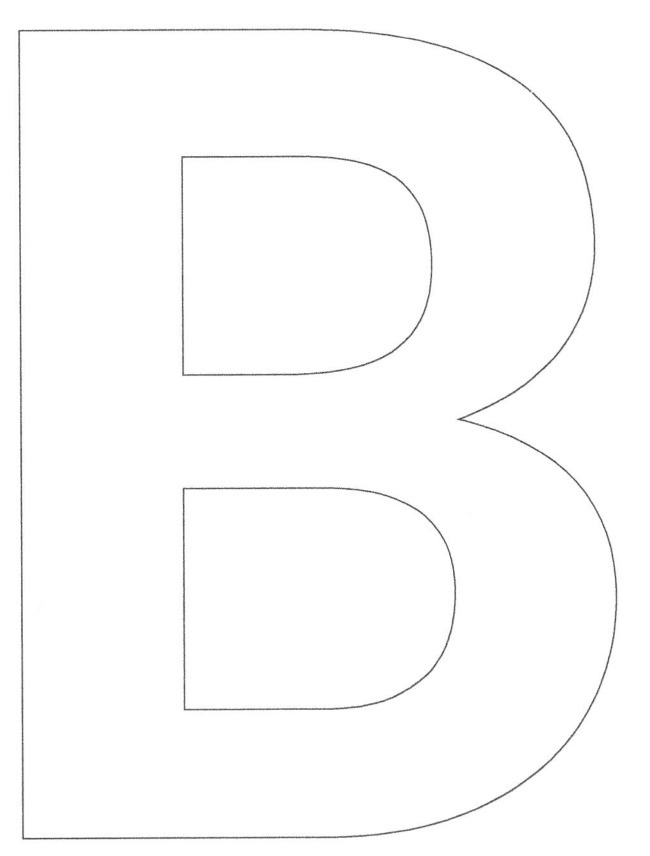

"Take a before photo to see where you are beginning. Vow to make this the last time you ever take one."

No more BEFORE photos

No more BEFORE photos

No more BEFORE photos

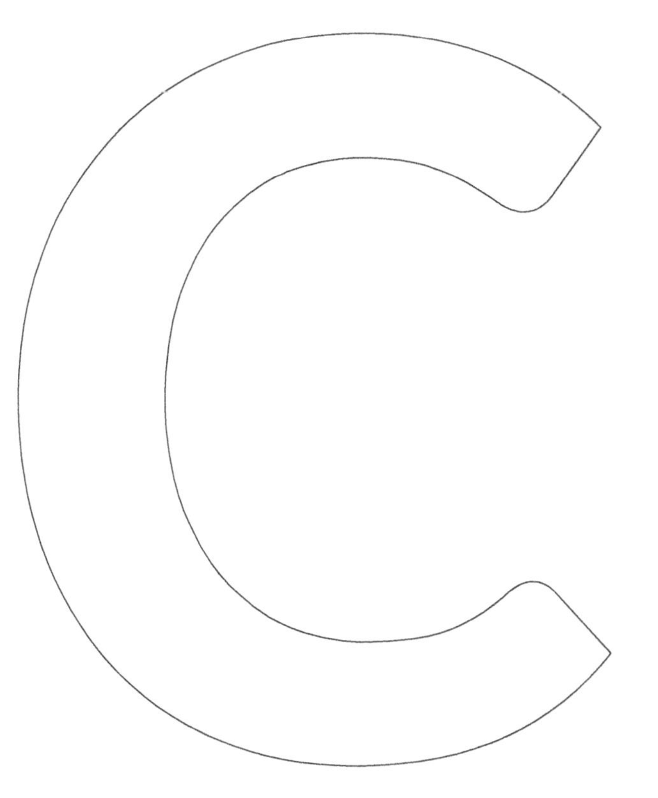

"No more wasting time. We've already done enough of that. Let's go."

C'MON with the C'MON
C'MON with the C'MON
C'MON with the C'MON

It's time for change. It's time for action. It's time to release the weight once and for all. That was my mindset last year. I weighed 239 pounds and had about a 40 inch waist. I knew that I needed to release the weight. I've always been active but I had a hard time getting both my exercise and nutrition dialed in at the same time. I knew what to do but my mindset wasn't where it needed to be.

One of the things that helped me successfully release 20 pounds and keep it off for almost a year was changing my thinking. I needed to flood my mind with positive thoughts.

I needed to remind myself that I could and would be successful releasing the weight once and for all. I was able to improve my health and fitness. I want you to be able to do the same thing.

I'm not saying that mindset is the only thing you will have to do to release the weight. Obviously, you will need to eat better and exercise. It will also help if you have some kind of support group. I have established an online support group. If you would like to be a part of it send me an email at benjaminleefitness@gmail.com. Are you ready to change? Are you ready to have a stronger mindset? Let's change that right now.

I've designed this coloring book to help you flood your mind with positive thoughts. Everyday during my transformation I would write out certain phrases multiple times in the morning telling myself what I was going to do. That's what I want you to do. But I've made it easier for you and a little more fun. I've already written out the motivational phrases for you, and now all you need to do is color them. Let's Color Our Way To Releasing The Weight!

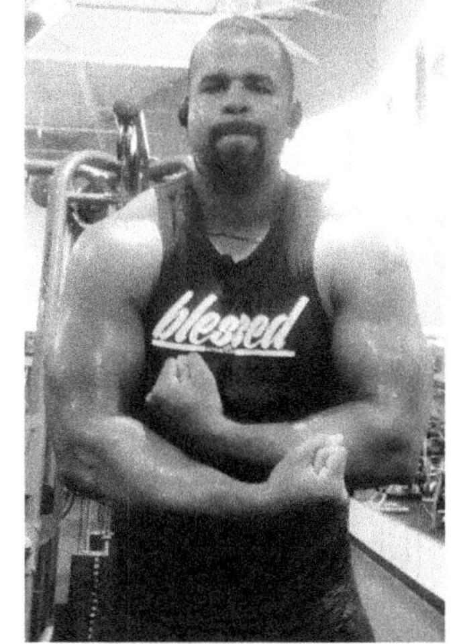

I believe in YOU!

Cmon with the Cmon. Let's go!

– Benjamin Lee
Follow Benjamin at benjaminleeonline.com
and benjaminlee.blog.

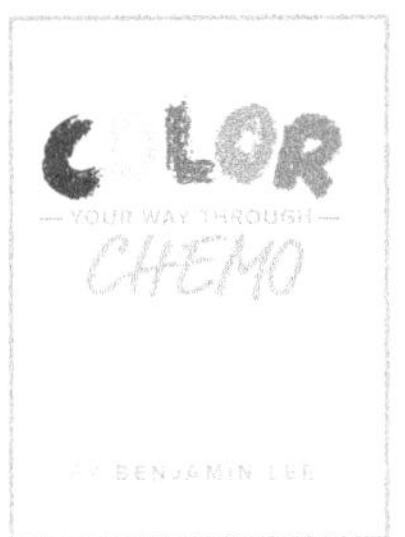

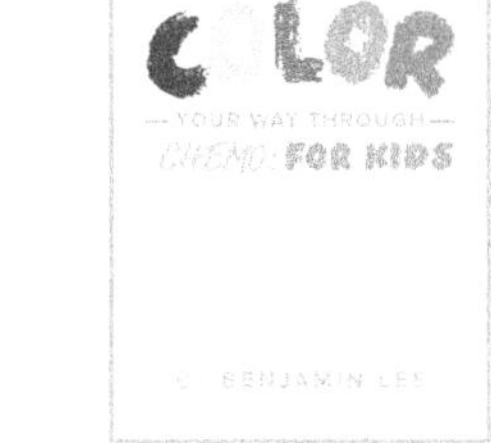

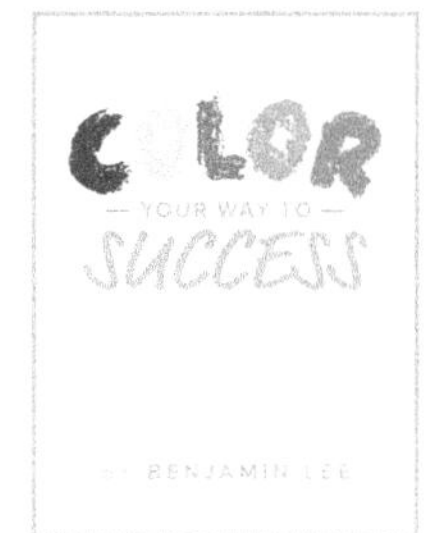

CYW THROUGH CHEMO   *CYW THROUGH CHEMO: FOR KIDS*   *CYW TO SUCCESS*

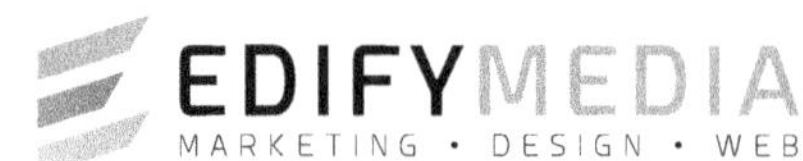

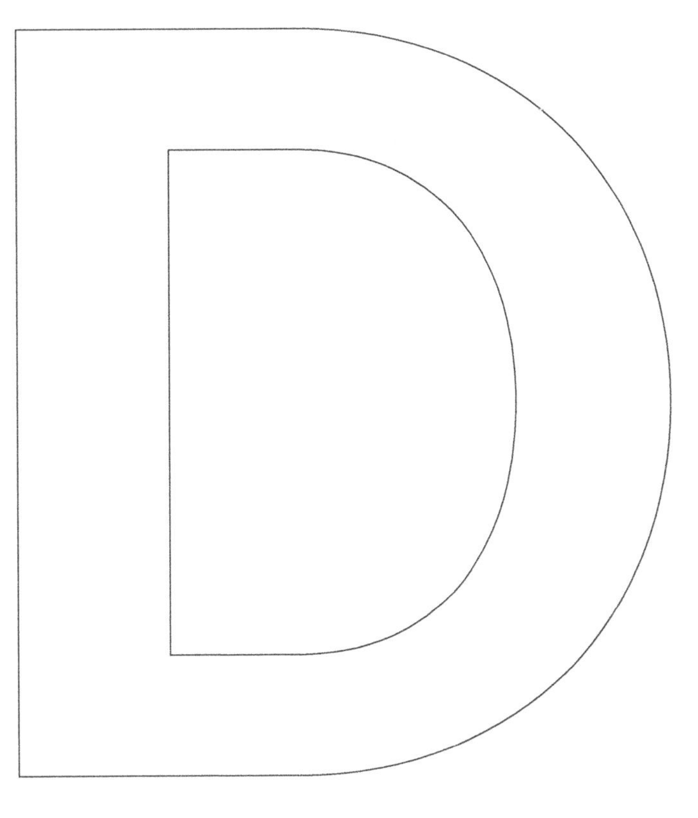

D

"This is all up to you. You get to decide the results you will have."

DECIDE and be DETERMINED

DECIDE and be DETERMINED

DECIDE and be DETERMINED

DECIDE and be DETERMINED

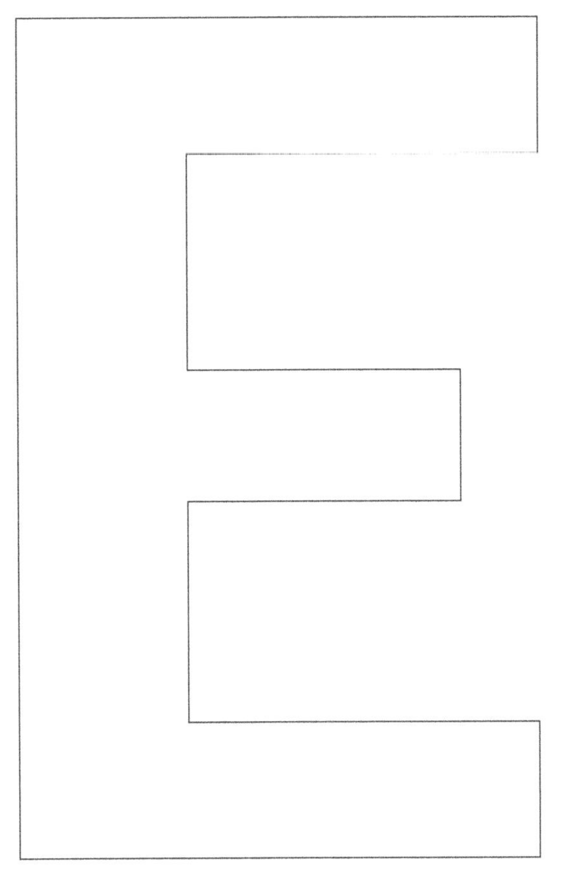

"This is a journey we're on. Enjoy every-day. You can do it."

ENJOY the process

ENJOY the process

ENJOY the process

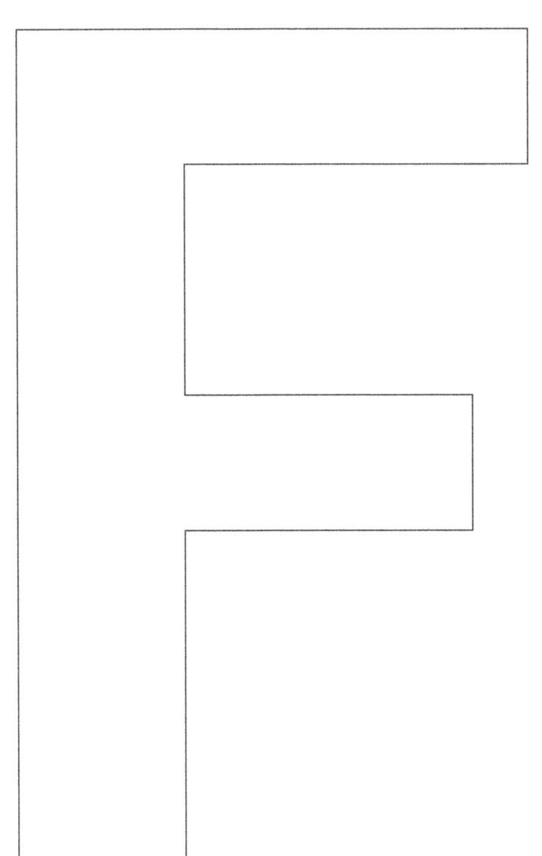

FOCUS and have FAITH

FOCUS and have FAITH

FOCUS and have FAITH

FOCUS and have FAITH

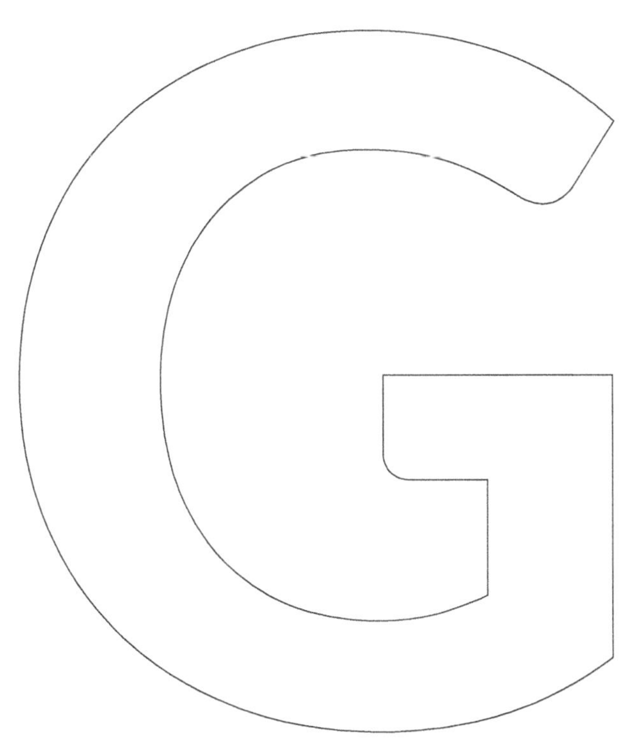

G

"This is about action. You either want it or you don't. Let's go."

GO, GO, GO

GO, GO, GO

GO, GO, GO

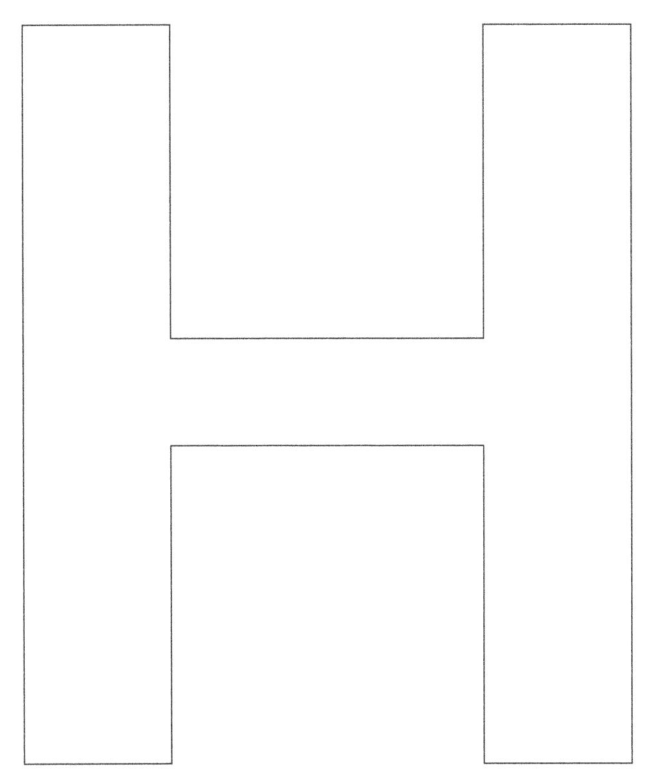

H

HIT the training HARD

HIT the training HARD

HIT the training HARD

HIT the training HARD

IGNORE the naysayers

IGNORE the naysayers

IGNORE the naysayers

IGNORE the naysayers

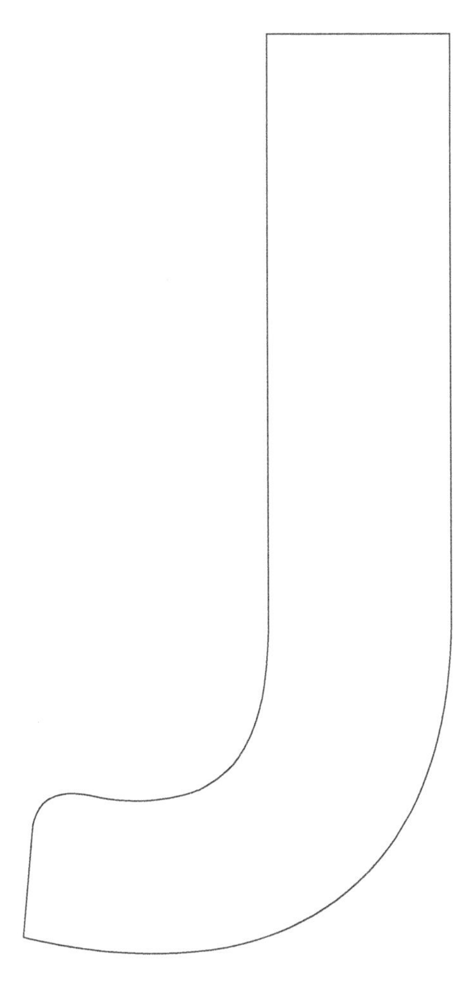

JUST keep going

JUST keep going

JUST keep going

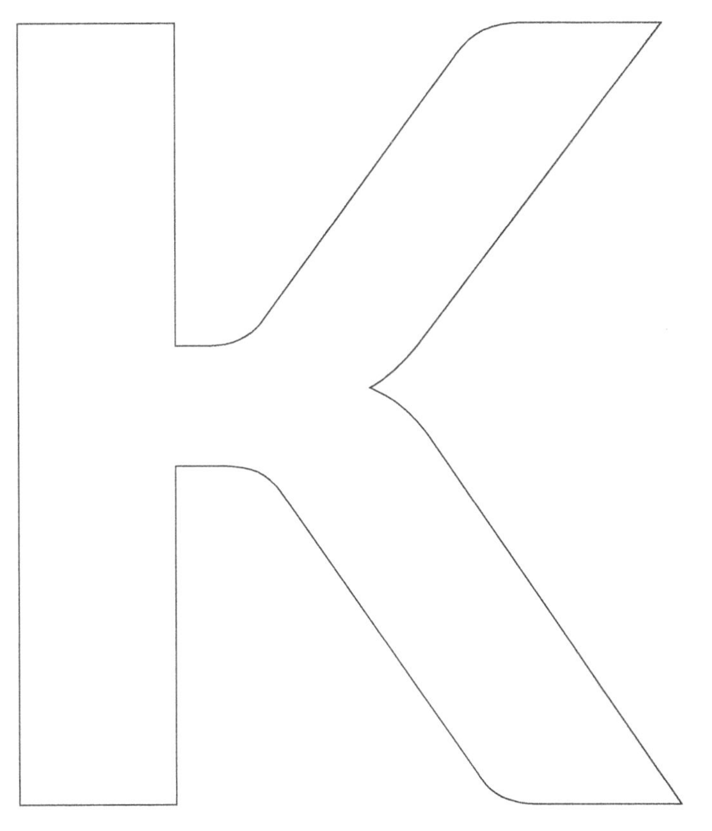

K

KEEP on KEEPING on

KEEP on KEEPING on

KEEP on KEEPING on

KEEP on KEEPING on

L

> *"Talk good to yourself. Quit beating yourself up so much."*

LOVE yourself

LOVE yourself

LOVE yourself

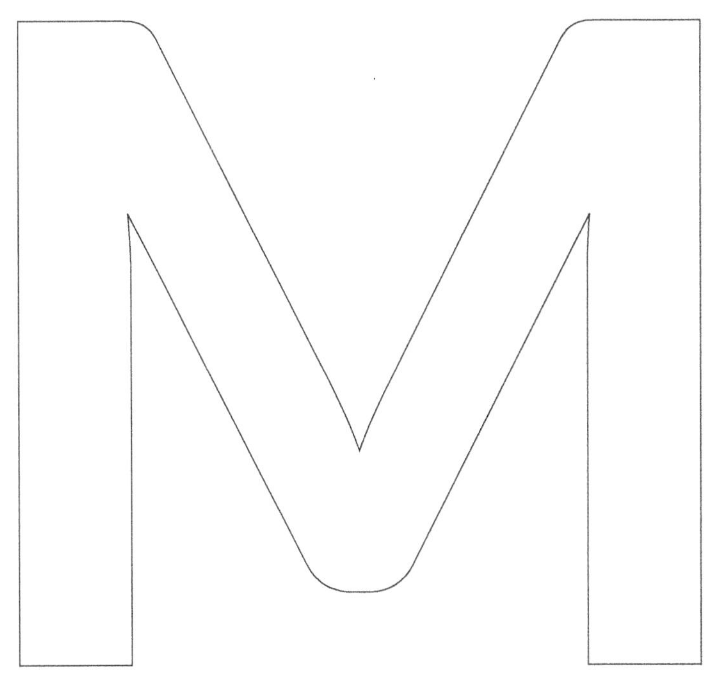

M

"*Do the simple things like preparing and planning your meals, exercising 5-6 days a week, and eating healthy. Results will follow.*"

MASTER the basics

MASTER the basics

MASTER the basics

MASTER the basics

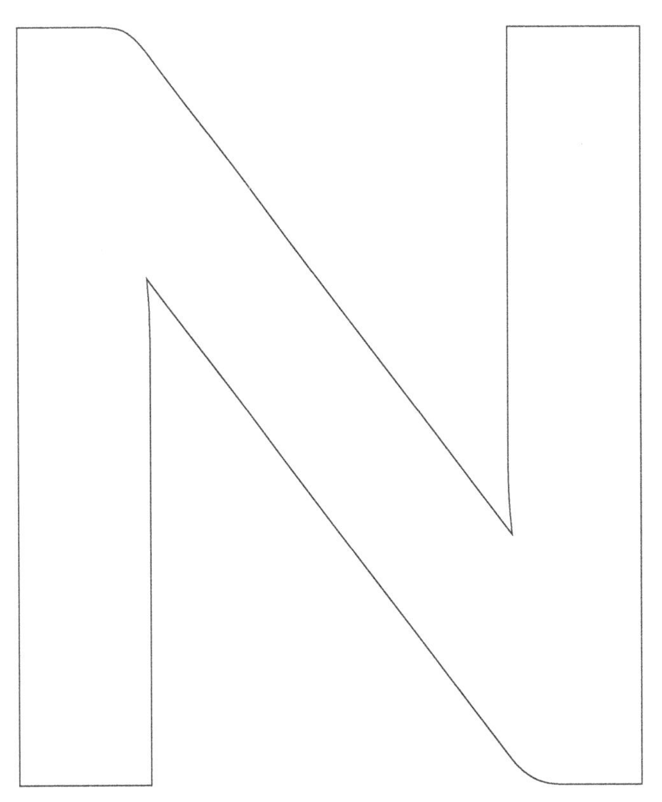

NEVER give up

NEVER give up

NEVER give up

"**Allow others to help you along the way. Receive compliments with a smile. You can't do this by yourself.**"

OPEN your heart to OTHERS

OPEN your heart to OTHERS

OPEN your heart to OTHERS

OPEN your heart to OTHERS

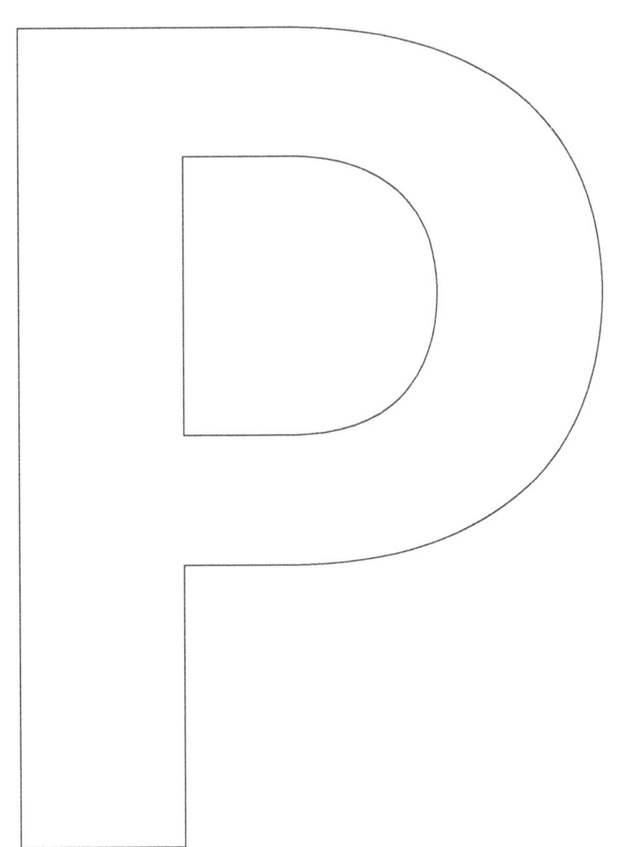

P

"Everyday is a step in the right direction." Just keep going."

It's about PROGRESS

It's about PROGRESS

It's about PROGRESS

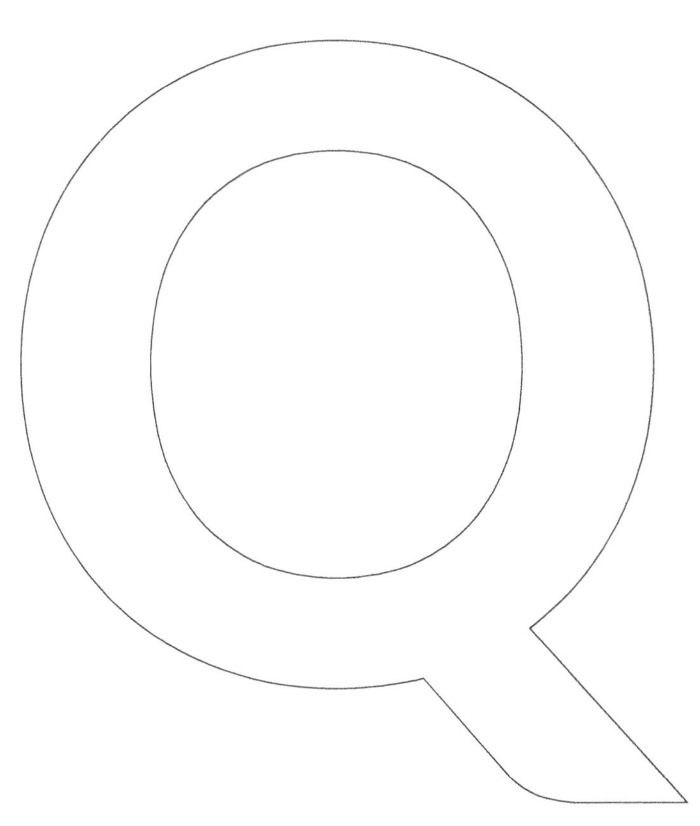

QUIT sabotaging yourself

QUIT sabotaging yourself

QUIT sabotaging yourself

QUIT sabotaging yourself

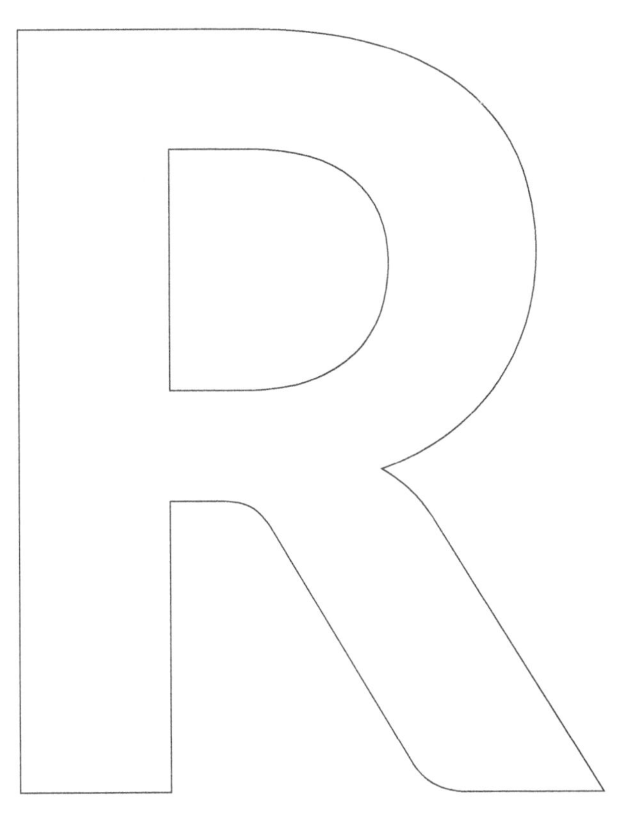

R

"Take the time to give yourself a pat on the back with the good work you've been doing."

REFLECT on the positives

REFLECT on the positives

REFLECT on the positives

REFLECT on the positives

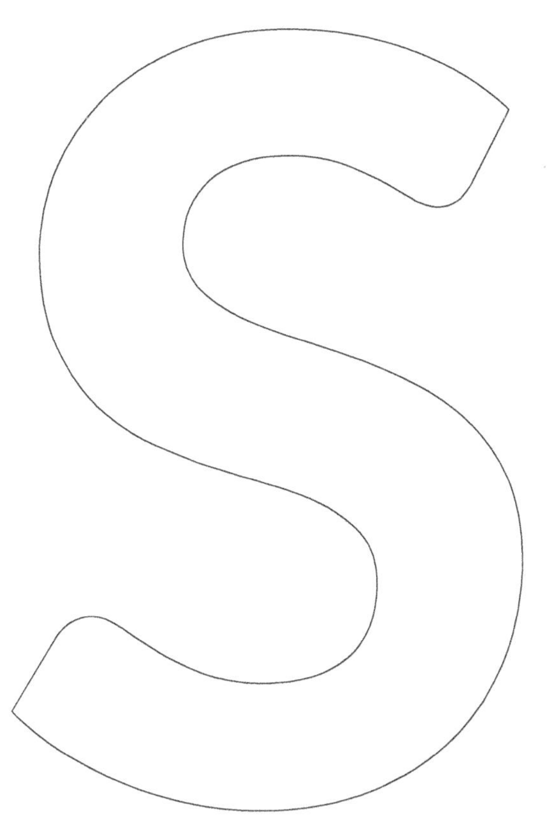

S

"Releasing the weight takes time. Be patient. We are not going after quick fixes."

SLOW and STEADY

SLOW and STEADY

SLOW and STEADY

T

> *"Think about where you want to be one year from now. It will take some time but you will get there."*

TAKE your TIME

TAKE your TIME

TAKE your TIME

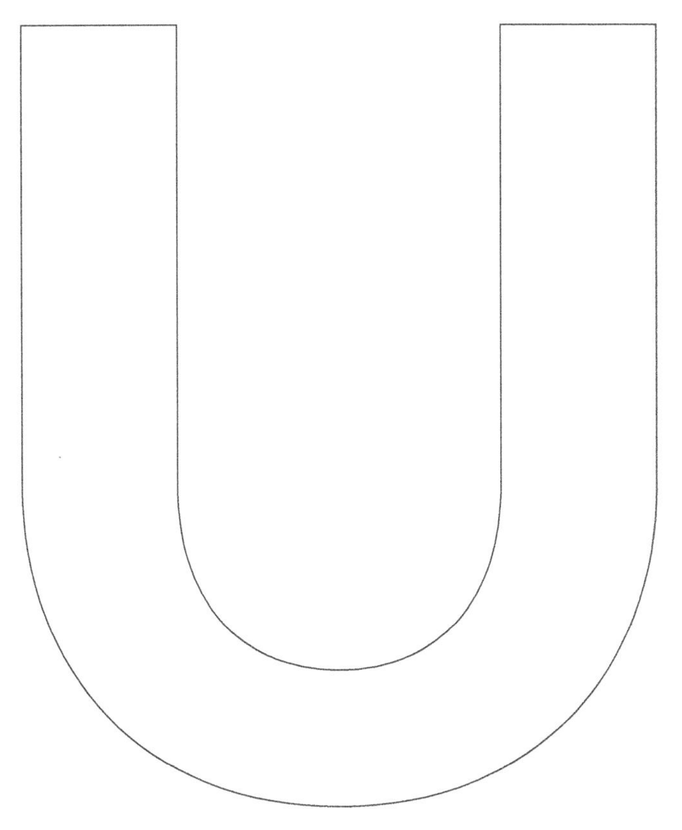

It's all about U

It's all about U

It's all about U

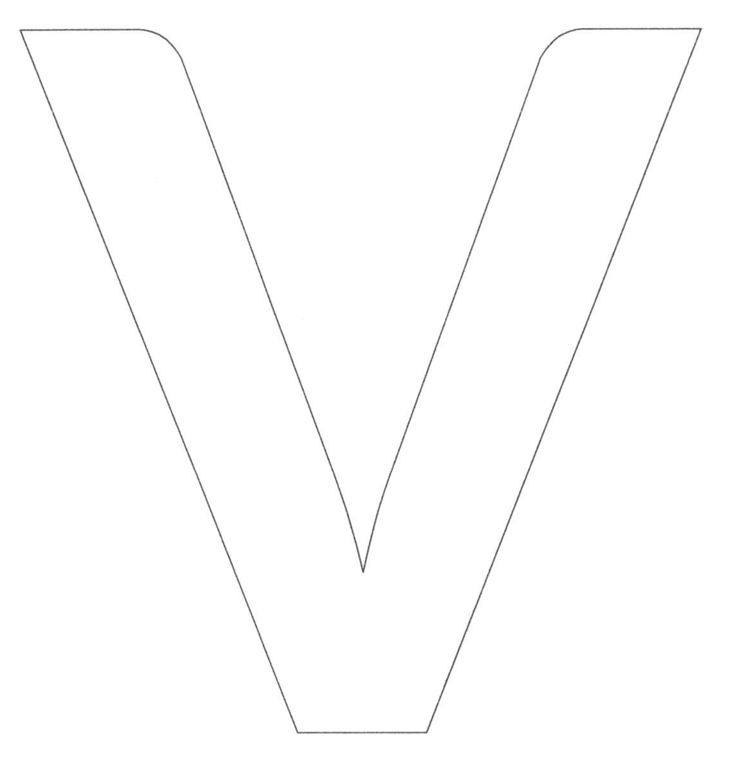

"Celebrate your victories. You've put in the hard work. You can do it."

VOICE your VICTORIES

VOICE your VICTORIES

VOICE your VICTORIES

VOICE your VICTORIES

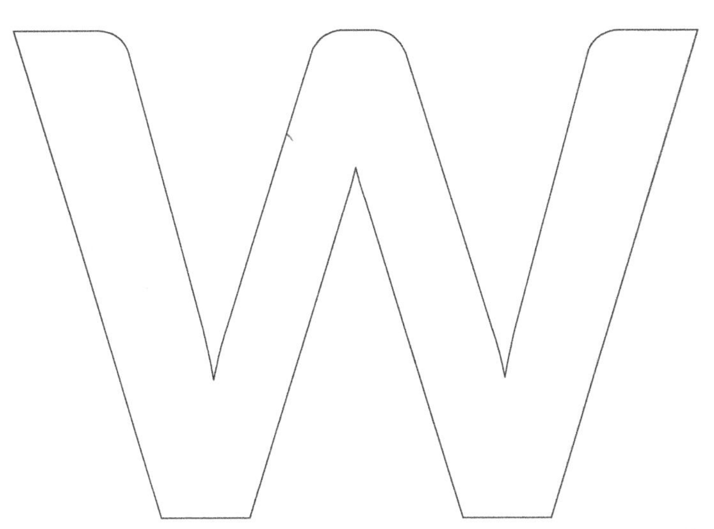

W

WAIT for the results

WAIT for the results

WAIT for the results

WAIT for the results

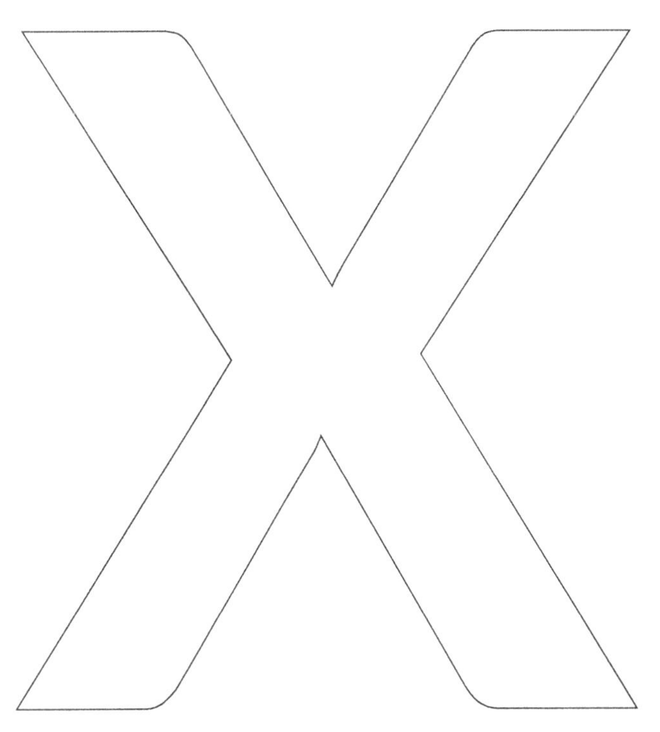

X

eXPECT eXCELLENT results

eXPECT eXCELLENT results

eXPECT eXCELLENT results

eXPECT eXCELLENT results

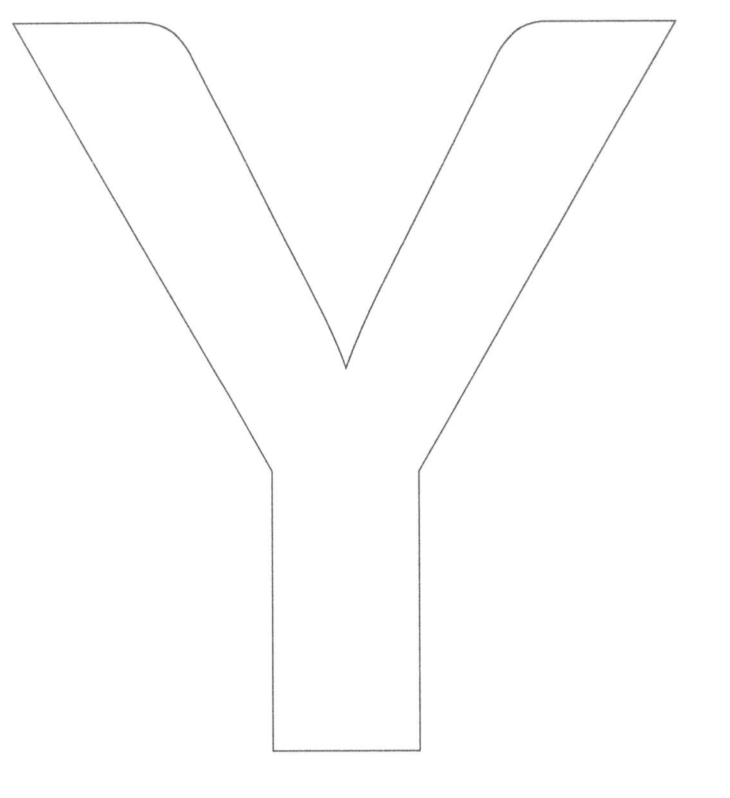

"A positive mindset is key. Fill your mind with good thoughts. Get rid of the junk."

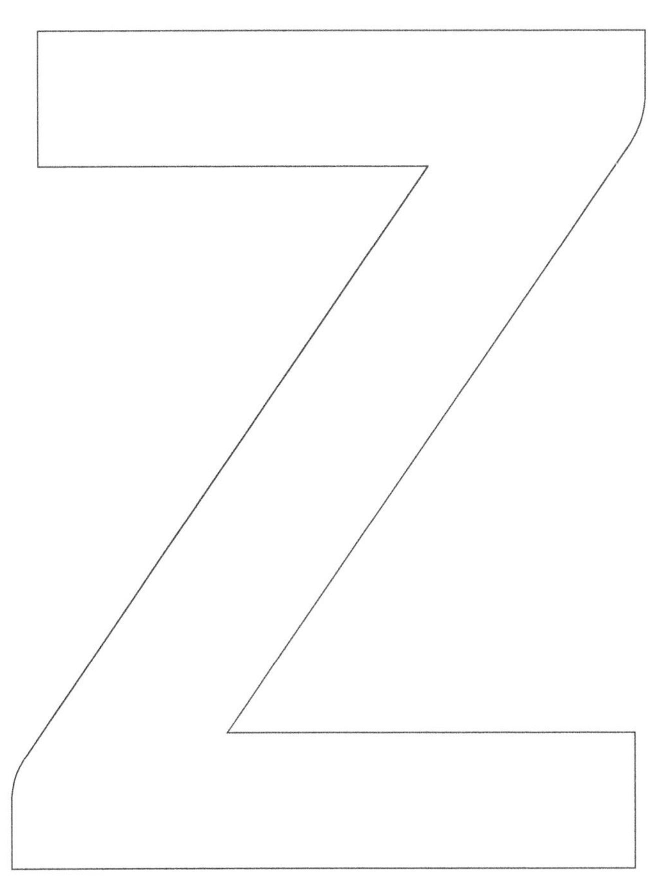

"You have to stay hungry. You have to want it. Let's go baby.

Stay ZEALOUS

Stay ZEALOUS

Stay ZEALOUS

www.ingramcontent.com/pod-product-compliance
Lightning Source LLC
Chambersburg PA
CBHW081249250726
48654CB00012B/1550